for Eleanor

about the author

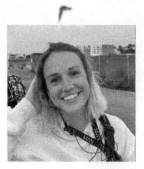

Lauren DeCamillo (she/her) is a 27 year old poet native to Ashtabula, Ohio who has called Columbus home for many years now.

Since her last published work in 2019, "*A Study in Controlled Heat*," the author earned her Bachelors of Arts degree in Arts Management from The Ohio State University and began a successful career in event operations.

Writing remains DeCamillo's primary passion and means of healing, but the resulting sophomore collection before you was birthed by more than four years of painstaking work and study to refine her craft.

for Eleanor

dedication

This collection is dedicated to Eleanor Paige DeCamillo. The Most Perfect Thing with a button nose.

Who poured into my life like a great flood, washing it all clean.

Who filled my weary soul with kicks and nursery rhymes and the promise of grins across chubby, giggling cheeks.

Who came into the world with little purple lips and shattered my heart before I ever got the chance to hold Her to its beating.

Eleanor, my precious, disappeared daughter, everything good in me, is You. Always.

for Eleanor

Cover Design by Theo Morrow.

for Eleanor

contents

for Eleanor

equator is an old friend ⇢ west ⇢
nymphs of colorado ⇢ after
nomadland ⇢ jimmy t's diner ⇢ the
night they blare billy strings on the
record player i drink all too much wine
and ruin everything

VII. *the burning cathedral 87*

ode to the water ⇢ i think about
this when i'm alone ⇢ this
summer ⇢ he makes coffee in
the mornings ⇢ castle rock (and
the death of it) ⇢ a love like god's

VIII. *for Eleanor 103*

The sun sets in Colorado and
Rises in Ohio ⇢ Someone said
'Ten Years' and I Missed You All
so terribly ⇢ At the Newport ⇢
On Spontaneity ⇢ The boy with a
chest like a swallow finds it ⇢ All
Things Go ⇢ The Earth Cracks
Open Again ⇢ for Eleanor

I. *exposition*

for Eleanor

for Eleanor

autumn's percussion
drips
from
the

trees
like
jazz

trickling
down

onto
snare.

Sets
the
pace

with
the
first

landing -
carries away

into the
beginning

of
the
end.

shall i

for Eleanor

learn

the love
song?

death's
delicate
dance -

handsome
contagion
coating

my green
lawn.

how lovely,
crisp -

shamelessly
trifling

in that
annual rot

which comes
without fail,

to suffocate

the
newly

breathing life.

for Eleanor

when it has to be enough

black SUV, packed beyond a view for the rear mirror-
another consolation prize for staying alive.
the gruesomest type of play acting
is a pretend revel in hanging by a thread.

thick air, greased handholds,
i long for something solid worth grabbing -
any morsel more appealing than giving in to gravity -
than the plunge into that deep. too dark to emerge
from again.

the Newness in the distance makes everything simpler.
i obsess - over the heroic speed with which It must be
captured,
and how It dulls, like fake gold rings
on unsuspecting green fingers.

it's a particular skill - spotting the sun's glint off a shiny,
horizon-lain little something -
all the while remaining too busy with the new chase to
notice any tarnish already building in these greedy
hands of mine.

even the great athletes only sprint so many times
before the legs wear beyond function.
even everest's climbers only survive so long in air that
thin.

so when the weary sets in, i return to the little blue
room in the little red corner of ohio.
pretend it doesn't feel like failure when mother
asks what i'd like for dinner.

for Eleanor

for Eleanor

before resurrection

go i to the pink horizon
way beyond the shore
far as limbs will carry me
til they can take no more

go i with the pulling tide
my ankles sucked beneath
this body to the far and wide
the salt that sweeps 'cross yonder reef

will strip these rattled bones of hide
will shred me piece by piece.
go i for one final ride
'till all the sound has ceased.

for Eleanor

for Eleanor

rise

the human world, yawning,
rears its head
without apology for the time
it took to rest.

a room in focus for the first time
since last night's weary,
placed gingerly over the eyes
like a new prescription.

and just like the sound of the creaking floor,
there are birds that cry through the brighter hours
which feel louder and more alive
at break of dawn.

sweep away the static,
uncover some crisp
wonder in the face
of the young, grinning day.

naked feet, breaching their familiar warmth,
meet the ground in silent strength
with which to shoulder the unexpected trials of the
waiting hours

and rise.

for Eleanor

for Eleanor

II. *all the wrong places*

for Eleanor

for Eleanor

the first

1. what could've been.

there is an overwhelming blue here.

sorrowful and longing.

the kind deep enough

only the ocean's craters know
it. a color hidden
with the soft of His upper lip
and all the other unrealized
fantasies i will never meet face to
face.

adolescent-almost-fumble,
a final one.
eyes so lure,
hands so push. young love
can only be tragic
if you let it

we will wonder for a while,
i suppose. a brooding,
unstruck match. grateful soon
enough that we've not made ash of ourselves.

2. what was.

simple restraint brings my childhood

to the great deep with her.

for Eleanor

like a good girl, she goes discreetly
to the ocean's bottom.
in the name of exploration,
to that big blue dark
where it is only appropriate to assume
neither of us find the surface in the end.

an adolescent
flush, more than we bargained.
children aren't supposed to
make choices like this. and we are-
children, after all. young love
will always be tragic
if you let it.

for years we run like wildfire.
making kindling of even the steal.
for years still we firefight.
rebuild. surviving charred
and sooty.

for Eleanor

the last

i didn't ask for
another love war.

no blood-stained dagger
on muddied ground.

in a more patient world,
maybe neither of us is a criminal.

on a day less consumed
by whose toe breached the line

first, i forgive
without checking the scoreboard.
and nobody bleeds.

for Eleanor

for Eleanor

a place where your pain isn't currency

there's nowhere i do not trade calloused hands for
upturned lips -
nowhere i do not blister my feet chasing butterflies

i suppose
if there were such a place
i would not need so many blood transfusions -

would not pass out pints to every person
that looked at me like a full dinner plate
and called this love

i suppose,
if there were such a place
my body might think itself more than just something to
open

might not insist on some value in the bruises and lack
of breath
might never have learned the conversion rates
of pain to pleasure to begin with

i suppose,
if there were such a place
i could leave the suture in until the thread falls out -

let the scar heal over
instead of convincing myself again
that there's always some price to pay.

for Eleanor

for Eleanor

pining

on particularly boring or late nights,
my mind winds its way back
to that violent and moving unlonesomeness
from which i swore abstinence long ago.

on the dark wooded roads
where You made poetry
of the bitter winter, i drink
the wine alone this time.

rewrite the story
until it's easier to forgive.
until we are Predator and
prey no longer. rewrite

until i'm primed again
for hunting. "ungrateful girl-
what kind of dreary life
would you live without Me

to come make all the pretty things
cold and complicated?"
and if i'm bored of this world
i've built without Your fickle, passioned cutting-

if it all scars over and leaves
my insides hollow,
well, what of me then,
but to cry out to an empty room?

for Eleanor

for Eleanor

temptation

i open the door
and again this town deafens me
with its silence.

for years, this Weapon into my side

reopen the wound, would You?
won't You remind me, the cold
lingering pain of abandon?

with every visit the line a little duller in the sand

washing slowly away -
forgetting who drew it in the first place,
and why.

as though i didn't swear upon it

like religion.
as though i didn't learn the heat of
Purgatory first hand

one hundred times over.

You still visit my dreams in apologies.
coaxing with seafoam eyes
erasing every vow i made

to myself.

for Eleanor

for Eleanor

relapse

i could make the drive in a blindfold.
right at the corner store
left onto bunker
start to finish
without a pothole stirred.

nine minutes flat. eight if it's late
enough that the streets have gone quiet -
usually it is.

like biblical prophecy,
damning comes with the partaking.
swatches of my skin, ripped
like cheap fabric, drying out

how crumbs do
on your mother's freshly vacuumed
floor. my body
pulls itself apart
trying to keep me from You.

i pretend this isn't a warning.

for Eleanor

for Eleanor

conception

nothing has been rose colored here in ages.
gray scale and flashes of violent
crimson. He wants

my wrists tied to the piano
in His childhood
room. to breathe life
to the puppet strings
tugging me already.

there is a threshold in which
His hand becomes my back,
that i've yet to dislodge,
for fear of the way a body binds
to the objects that impale it.

sometimes i call this
piercing love. name
the Captor a part of me
until His release. and carry
on into the gray.

for Eleanor

,

for Eleanor

III. (s)mother

for Eleanor

for Eleanor

mosquito

day 27
the stillwater source-
usual place to lay. my
morning, strange. bloodless.

day 28
the larva molts. my
body stagnant, no shedding.
breed fear with insect.

day 29
pupa splits Her skin.
nothing in me opens still.
She grows. comes hunting.

day 30
cannot go ignored.
two pink lines, She finds a feast.
and i drain to Her.

for Eleanor

for Eleanor

Poppyseed II

it's a wonder - something so small ripping the universe
apart. today
i have more faith in the big bang than ever.

decisions, so uncomplicated
when hypothetical.
in the mock-up, i disappear

this inconvenience
with the timely ease
of my annual dental cleaning.

so simple, until it isn't.
until they're calling me back to the room
to look at timelines and tiny figurines
and simplicity, that beautiful illusionist,

abandons her curtain call. i pretend not to
notice when mrs small-town-so-and-so sees me
there, undereyes salt-stained,
lids swollen with doubt.

pieces of a Poppyseed tearing through my insides like
shrapnel.

for Eleanor

for Eleanor

mother

Accident sleeps
in my bed. i tuck Her in
like porcelain. or
paper doll.
i mother Accident like Purpose.
driven fateful into swaddle and

rocking chair. incubate
this new Fear and extinguish
the elder.
She and i the same,
i think. bursting forth and

helpless.
each a late night, wailing
warm body, bewildered gaze.
each uncovering love for the
first time.

for Eleanor

smother

misery sleeps
in my bed. i tuck her in
like an old friend. or
a child.
mother misery like my First Born
should my First Born have breathed a breath

to begin with. suffocate
my real Child in lieu of
this vapid one.
love them both the same,
i think. each of them a death

sentence.
each so integral in
pulling apart my ribs.
only one i have the gall to
smother.

for Eleanor

on god

my sister says, *i will be an aunt either way.*
says *God plans everything.*

this is meant to be helpful
but it is robbery.

and if my body is its' own to worship
she is a liar.

for Eleanor

for Eleanor

IV. the change and its quiet

for Eleanor

for Eleanor

mother II

maybe, were i better,
i'd say the day i decided on You
the sky stopped falling.

that all stood perfectly still which hadn't before, and
there was tranquility and untainted air, and that hulking
roof with all its water quit pouring down through the
gaping holes i'd left.

maybe, were i better,
the shelter would've been in place
from the very start -

no need for newfound patchwork skill on the shingles.
but two hands which fail for the sake of themselves
can make the labor of a village look simple
under the right conditions.

new life - in the word mother. a sniveling
child of chaos turned to peace
on behalf of that smaller, more helpless little
Love growing inside of me.

in time, for You my dear,
i will tie back together
all of the chasms in the sky.

for Eleanor

for Eleanor

a long quiet lays in this place
where all that I touch
is soft and small enough for the palm of my hand.

where every moment is purposeful,
from my love,
for My Love,
I craft bone and tissue.
I craft nothing else.

where self discipline belongs not to Me alone,
I exercise in the mornings.

where sadness belongs not to Me alone,
I paint the world yellow.

where fear belongs to both of Us,
I am athena..

where the hunt belongs to both of Us,
I am single target.
skilled archer. trained eye.

where My pining is Hers too,
he can not find Me here.

where My restless is Hers too,
I tuck myself in early - safe and warm.

autumn belongs to the both of Us -
the tranquil beauty of rebirth
while the fallen leaves die.

for Eleanor

i think about writing this - on that day by the lake, while
loved ones bathe Us in promise
and the sound of crinkling leaves soothes this steady
mothers' worry of mine,

but there is no creative revolution in peace.
it just is.
and We live like this the whole way through.

for Eleanor

V. please stop sending flowers

for Eleanor

for Eleanor

hush - the end of a dance

dance in the hush hush
surround sound melodies all
rest play crescendo

one Voice which carries
crisp through the warbling 'till the
movement - - stops

We wake together
retire together We
dance in the hush hush

We take nutrients
and power naps. take the blame
and the pedestal.

prepare for something
it's Me i think my exit
from the muffled dark

dance in the hush hush
cramped in the hush - it must
be about that time

a gentle waltz but
Voice really does not feel my
footsteps - waiver?

hear Me imploding?
my - lungs - -
running - - dry

for Eleanor

- Voice - cannot
feel as - - I'm thrashing?
- pleading - -

wriggle in the hush
music - wanes powerless
 - - - goodbye

train - - vanish
into tunnel -
- - outro fades

for Eleanor

"i'm sorry"

i am a panic
in the lightning.
hurricane's eye meets mine, a blind
date too late to cancel.

she reassures, *'did you hear that?'*

but i see the trees contorting.

'She's just hiding. i'll get someone else.'

the roof buckles.

'let's get some more jelly on there. a little '

cold air.

'pressure.'

shattered windows.

wading in vain, the blue wall grows.
the little picture doesn't move
and doesn't move
and doesn't move.

i hold my breath.
two words come with the crack of her voice.

and the water,
the water takes me.

for Eleanor

for Eleanor

(la)maze

i hear her moaning from the hallway.
from the sixth floor.
from the other side of the city.

i am in a place where
none of this has happened yet.
a dimly lit lamaze room with purple carpet and a

> bathroom
> too far to reach.
> only a couple of steps, if she could just get

'up. that's right,
have your partner lift up on that towel and
you should feel the-'

> retching.
> the peak and the screams.
> *'no!'* she can't

'breathe. yes!
picture something, a focal point.' i see paint.
purple drip

into blue
drip into
purple drip into

> red
> on the tile floor and
> the stench of

for Eleanor

a vanilla candle
burning in the corner,
it's

                                        acrid, iron
                          pervading the space.
the knuckles of some non-mother's ghost around the
                                          railing.

the woman at my feet
with her warm smile and cascading
strawberry blonde

                                    bun crouches,
                                    arms out and
                  i-no, the ghost-

                                  the ghost wails.
                                  'there's no more

divine purpose here.'
the thought of that crying infant in your arms. the best
part about her tears is that you are exactly what -'

                              couldn't save Her.
and no matter how long you hold Her cold little body,
                        the tears will not come.

for Eleanor

when i wake

i don't really wake.
this room is nightmare
the blood smell too strong
for any other kind of
dream. dead and somehow the heart
revives me without beating.

when i wake

my sister holds Her.
i feel guilty. worry She's
too heavy. where did
i think stillborns went after
the screaming? how can she bear
to touch my cold dead Daydream?

when i wake

"all that fentanyl"
the nurses say it over
"we gave her all that fent-"

when i wake

they say i need to
pee. at minimum, sit up.
i, crash test dummy.
they lift like there's no blood to
lose. like i won't faint while they
reset the accident-

when i wake

for Eleanor

"i'm going to press-"

"the social worker wants-"

"we're just gonna change-"

    when i wake

my mother stirs. no
one is sleeping if i'm not.
i must be because
She is. Eleanor. sleeping
just for now. just, tired.
"need anything?" *nothing you can give me.*

    when i wake

i'll call the "reason for visit"
night terrors. the
nurse will give a strange look. take the
payment. call the doctor.

this time, the ultrasound will move.

for Eleanor

arrangements: a non-poem from the depths of grief

back seat
white building
square sign
parking lot
back door
locked door
    too early.

back seat

man
tall man
mustache
door
handshake
    don't cry.

hallway
                            "on the right"
chair
    wrong chair.
    center chair.
condolences
                                    "thank you"
                          "well then…"
full name
    don't cry.
                          "birth date"
                                    "11/14/19"
                        "death date?"

for Eleanor

"11/14/19"

"right, i'm-"

"don't worry
about it."

hospital
doctor

"father?"

"irrelevant."

"well-"

"uninvolved."

"ok."

service size

"service type?"

"well i was
thinking
cremation."

"alright

so this would be the urn."

"that small?"

"well

you don't get much back."

jesus.

"right.

maybe burial."

"we'll have to talk plots.
do you have family plots?
or you can always purchase
one."

for Eleanor

"ok cremation."

"cremation?"

"um

yeah."

"you're sure?"

no.

"sure."

"obituary?"

"can i email
you?"

"of course, of course
but
quickly?"

right

"yeah of
course, right
away."

"and um
the father knows?"

"yes."

"and you're certain he's-"

"yes."

paperwork
low ink
new pen
small talk
stomach ache
paperwork

"and a date?"

oh right.
don't puke.

for Eleanor

"let me check
my calendar."

cell phone
unlock

"you'll want to find a minister
too"

"right"

right...
cell phone
cell phone?
oh, calendar
where's the app
calendar.
scroll
of course
empty.

"saturday?"
"saturday should work.

i can get someone from almost
any religion."

"religion?"
"to speak."

oh, right.

"jewish?
catholic?"

guess i'll call the guy from my old church

"can i uh
can i just tell
you in the
email?"

for Eleanor

"no problem.
no problem at all.

okay well..."
right.
more condolences
stand
maroon carpet
hallway
more hallway

"this will be the room but
someone's in there now."
say something.
nod
good enough.
hallway
back door
condolences
don't cry,

"thank you"
don't puke.
outside
back seat
shut door

release.

i must have woken up by now.

for Eleanor

for Eleanor

please stop sending flowers

the doorbell bites with the dull of my grandmother's
pruning shears.
another day, another
empty-faced delivery
boy carving chasm into my stomach.

who decided to sooth
tears with an artform
that inevitably
causes the eyes to water?

why is the consolation
for death
always just another
dying thing?

the obligatory funeral invite
in too much
lipstick calls them,
'a tribute to her beauty.'

for some unknown reason
i do not ask her
why then, anyone insisted that
the flowers *too* be ripped from
roots that fed them into bloom.

after the service
my dining room boasts
greenery and good intentions.

i stare at the petals

for Eleanor

and bleed
until every last one falls.

VI. in the after

for Eleanor

for Eleanor

after the sobbing and bleeding

after the hand holding and the hospital food -
the muddled sorrys and thank yous

after the weird branded souvenirs from strangers and
wilted flowers and flavorless casseroles,
and flavorless everything else -

after the smug stench of convenience dripping from
his pores, masked in the cheap cologne of sympathy -
the card signed by his mother and it's eerily similar
scent -

after the dressing and redressing -
the prescription drugs - the surgery and the mesh
underwear -

after the other drugs, taken privately, masked in red
wine, grief and low tolerance -

after the hours of mind numbing- sleep, television, the
same music videos on repeat, the coloring books and
novels and journal entries and anything to keep from
going mad with sorrow -

i can't sleep in that bedroom anymore.

not with Her initials on the wall
not with the tiny clothes hangers and the pastel
shelving
and the purple rocking chair.

not with the empty crib

for Eleanor

and the pink teddy bear urn
and the bloody sweater from its sole wear on one little
cold body.

complacency here is a death sentence.
as soon as the pain is dull enough,
i turn west in the name of survival
and try to convince myself that anything at all is holy.

for Eleanor

run

every middle-aged woman in the airport is your
mother
every young woman is her daughter
and every little girl, is
Mine.

every dirty blonde - untamed curls - sapphire eyes
looks like coming home,
and i am vagabond. dirty
fingernails, train car cold and false freedom.
today, i run without consequence.

please, tell me,
now that i've lost Her,
must i plunge into the depths of you again?

for Eleanor

for Eleanor

on writing, or lack thereof

darling, scandalous page
gazing at me
like a radiant woman
longing for touch -
i fear i don't know
how to love you anymore.

too afraid for the
bleeding ink -
and the silhouette it paints
when i give it the power to.

how do i love you and also myself?
how do i stain you and not brand this skin
with some gaping scar
i'll look back on, calling it youth and toil?

this curse, heavy with the hunger
to create - rife with shame
for the sound of honesty's written word
dripping from my pen.

once they've seen my pulsing heart
spray gore across
the crisp white paper,
how can any stranger love me then?

when i,
fitted with loyalty to this
weary mind and body,
am not so impressed with me either.

for Eleanor

for Eleanor

the equator is an old friend

both home and pioneer
both hard work
and slow deep breaths of the buddha
unsung hero of the unafraid

and everything here is medicine.
the salt of the air
the song of the crashing seafoam.
blood red faces flush with the sun's washing

and there's the equator-
strong enough to hold the whole earth in her arms
and still have more to give

for Peggy

for Eleanor

for Eleanor

west

the world unfolds in front of me for the first time,
Eleanor -
the way kerouac talked about
the red west of his youth.

the plains really do roll and roll.
this big vast ocean of sky and grain and hollow.
 so empty, you've no choice
but to think about

everything you ever thought or did
or thought about doing -
and everybody you ever loved
or never had the chance to,

and every view you ever saw,
sprawled out
like a novel that's been read so much
its binding is tired.

i brought this typewriter
as far as my wallet would take the two of us
nothing i wrote was
good enough.

instead i left your name carved into every beautiful
thing that would take its shape.
nothing suffices to fill this void.
i keep trying anyway.

for Eleanor

for Eleanor

nymphs of colorado

move in day is ascension,
wrestling dogs on a ragged carpet,
meat pie in the hands of a proud, young,
stoned woman at the staircase helm -

a trophy of welcome home in thrifted jeans
and a smile like the first time you saw the color yellow.
she makes warm of this place
better than the light cutting through the split-level
windows.

her best friend, in the corner under the canopy,
always burning her sadness, blowing it away
into smoke clouds that bend the mirrored room.
laughter contagious in an oversized t-shirt.

thud of a duffle on the stained floor,
ten tons off this heavy chest and its labored breathing.
finally, a place to settle, among the other nymphs
looking for answers somewhere in the foothills.

maybe i *will* survive in the end.

for Eleanor

for Eleanor

after nomadland

what is she searching for,
the woman who doesn't know how to stay?
among those trees - trunks like houses,
light catching just right on the dew -

everybody dies or goes.
she can feel herself doing the same-
slowly. wrinkles deeper
each day in the scratches of the campground mirror.

this life's careless hourglass
with all its empty air.
this empty air and all the love she could fill it with
if only she had the time -

this time she'd find it. the answer -
that makes the splintered glass glisten.
that paints the grieving clouds' silver outlines
as they cry beauty and pain

into the wide, fickle world.

for Eleanor

for Eleanor

jimmy t's diner

the man in the diner says, 'i'm off to meet the day again"
and bids his friends adieu with the kind of familiarity
owned only by gray men in places like this.

these four trusty walls and this black coffee
and shannon with her loud mouth making scrambled
eggs on the other side of the counter even on the most
glum of mornings at 8 o'clock sharp.

8 o'clock sharp when the man is in his stool,
third from the end with the little rip in the seam right on
the edge
and it doesn't need the man's name on it, for it is
marked with the wear of the years.

and everyone here knows his name and his stool
anyhow.
even the drifting customers who come in for their hot
cakes every couple of weeks
and don't speak to anybody- feel a little bit of home

when they see the newspaper
tucked so casually in the crook of the man's arm.
he wonders if they, in their silence, are also
quite so painfully lonely.

for Eleanor

for Eleanor

the night they blare billy strings on the record player i drink all too much wine and ruin everything

searching for the same story over
like a lost home vhs tape.
precious memories stamped out.

recorded over. my grappling
for nostalgia is helpless, save
from recreating the moment somehow.

cuts never deep enough.
a master at reasons to do it again -
from another angle. i ask my keeper when

she will free me and the mirror cracks. we do another
take. this time in the quiet mountains.
in the solace of horsetooth rock

and her willing trees, bending
to build safety from
the sun. i light it all aflame

in the name of what could've been.
no goodbyes.
daybreak coming up in the windshield.

i've gotten so good at packing the car.

for Eleanor

for Eleanor

VII. *the burning cathedral*

for Eleanor

for Eleanor

ode to the water

at long last, an apology for all the hours spent writing
you wicked.
what shame
to blame the tides for following the moon.
what fear
not to know where the thrashing leads-
to ponder where the deep blue carries you after it's
had its fill.

o water, i have found it
and it is beautiful.

a simple shore
welcomes all my weathered glass -
calls it cathedral.

and if i am the shatter,
if i am the color
raining through the ceiling,
he is the stone. the iron. the
certainty
that keeps it all
from crumbling in the storm.

i collage myself into his steady
he concretes his arms around the mosaic of me
we do not need choirs here -
or priests or spectacle.

slow dancing to the sound of the simple echo -
two voices, four footsteps
and praise.

for Eleanor

for Eleanor

i think about this when i'm alone

the light of your hair-fall in my eyes
when we collapse, too caught up to make the bed.
i could swear this room was clean before

you arrived, but that was months ago.
no, days.
or hours? yes, just hours.

and i'm unsure
whether the clean will feel right ever again
if it comes with the absence

of your fingertips tracing firework
into my skin. your mouth breathing explosions
into a quiet crackle
that fades out each time You go.
don't.

yo, okay?
let's neither of us go?
ever?

for Eleanor

for Eleanor

this summer

is the heat i swore against -

that wants for nothing and so
holds, tight and sweating
with no plans to part.

the heat that turns in early-
charcuterie and a glass of wine.

my restless overflows so heavy you can taste it, like
liquor on the breath, wondering
where i go in my quiet
and how far it is away from you.

for Eleanor

for Eleanor

he makes coffee in the mornings

at dawn,
the song of a dark
roast, jostled from its sleepy
container.

just hardly different
from the light
patter of rain
beyond the kitchen window.

it is a simple thing.
patient and slow, he cranks
the cherry wood handle,
waiting for the teapot's whistle.

beans splitting
ever so politely. falling
in line to rustle
steady through the blades.

hour-glassing themselves
into the vessel below.
white knuckled and grinning
for the water's warmth.

a bright new
aroma permeates the room
with their bathing

and in this lovely,
intimate quiet,
we drink.

for Eleanor

for Eleanor

Castle rock (and the death of it)

i fall in love with you
every single day
arms stretched like a prayer
in the dark of the 6:30 alarm,
preparing to soldier away
into a world that i still haven't quite mastered

storms roll through
like clockwork in the early afternoon
to feed the thirsty brush,
and send the climbers scurrying
down from their windy peaks,
while the sun coats most of our other hours

on your off days,
it's all tan lines
and freckles
and pool chairs
and books on the political climate.

there was that new seltzer brand
that blew up that summer
and the caffeine bars we ate
instead of lunch or breakfast
and the dogs on the patio - having gotten lost there
or just stopping by with their owners to say hello

there was the morning coffee
in the sharp balcony air
and the certainty of "it's going to be okay" in your voice
when i am pale and lifeless
and feel oh so burdensome again

for Eleanor

and the pouch of color-coded clips
i snap into my hair each day
and the learning to buzz yours for you
while the barber shops are closed
and the sunscreen applied to keep your scalp from
burning

there's the retiring home, still damp from the pool,
into the showers steam
where your lashes and brows darken,
water running down high cheekbones
and the gentle rinse of soap
from the tattoo on your right shoulder blade

there's the getting high and dancing
- leon bridges in the kitchen
and the silly little video games during the rain
or the forest fires that kept us inside so often

and the cruise to the grocery store, where you are so
thoughtful over every item
and i am so impatient that i have no choice but to make
light of it

there's the perfect little italian spot around the corner
with the buffalo pizza you love so much, (so we order it
every time)

and the plants we kept alive almost that whole
summer before they were
tumbled by the careless wind over and over, or before
the parasites took up real estate there

for Eleanor

and there's this way i play it all over -
like a cargo ship leaving the shore
as it sails straight away into the distance -
the thing we built,
once too massive to fathom,
shrinking smaller and smaller each time i glance back
at the sea

and the way you left the shoreline without turning your
eyes, even once, to watch it go.

for Eleanor

for Eleanor

a love like god's

we built our world
how god did.
self-righteous.
too quickly to attend to

the nuance
that would tear this
beautiful thing apart
from itself eventually.

looked down upon it.
called it good.

lately i wonder
if the feeling we named love
is ever anything more
than prolonged Infatuation.

didn't the bible say
"god loves his children"?
the ones he granted free will
and then damned for using it.

shook like
an etch-a-sketch when
they spent too long disobeying.
and weren't they perfect at first?

a fascination
that they could be so
unlike him

for Eleanor

and yet still so pretty.

didn't i claim to love you too,
just the same?
wasn't your steady
my favorite thing for a while?

the presumed intention in a stoic face
the tempered patience -
certainty in every footstep,
the routine, like clockwork.

didn't i praise you
for being mountain
and so quickly grow tired
of your massive unmoving?

and didn't you love me too,
you thought?
watch the chaos take hold
and start to believe in anarchy?

the way anything but passion
was just too heavy.
incapable of standing still.
hand-picked flower petals strewn across your sparkling
floor.

didn't you rave about
the color i splashed on the walls,
just before your nausea
over the mess it made?

for Eleanor

VIII. *for Eleanor*

for Eleanor

The sun sets in Colorado and Rises in Ohio

and still I haven't a single answer to any big life lessons
- those mysteries of death and the heart that go so
pitifully unsolved

at dawn on the fourteen thousand foot summits where
all the lost people have come hunting for them.

Beneath the lackluster Columbus sky,
a cornucopia - intricately woven and captivating not so
long ago - frays into ruin.

Another storm barreling through the midwest air,
tearing apart a brilliant day like its warmth was nothing
to begin with.

How many lashings must one take at the hands of the
universe before it's had its fill?

How much decay must one feed the soil before they've
fertilized the garden enough that the tired buds might
bloom?

I tell my partner that I am so much compost. That I am
the stench of all the lessons, and none of the color in
the flower petals anymore. He - has never been
swayed by my metaphors, really.

Has never felt his flesh melt away into the dirt - which
is to say he has never lost anything he loved -

which is all to say, I suppose, that I do wonder if maybe
he has not ever loved to begin with.

for Eleanor

It is the year's first honest heat and the sun prepares for
rest once more.
I am another day older - hardly any wiser.

It is springtime,
and the bright, timid chime of new keys,
and the fresh white of a canvas.

I weep
into the garden bed that is Me.
Expectant and patient,
watching as the green peaks through.

for Eleanor

Someone said 'Ten Years' and I Missed You All so Terribly

The thought of it jolting me,
I wind my way to the brick path by the library.
Wide and true -
healthy green so carefully manicured around it.

So lush and thoughtful.
Recalling those tender days in early fall- in late spring-
matting that same lawn with sport and relaxation.
And don't I feel so old in this place now?

Even on the holiday,
when most of the young, spry faces
abandon it for their short taste of freedom,
I ponder every little piece -

and whether it was here then,
and the promises we made each other
in overcrowded rooms amidst cheap liquor bottles or
dining hall food.

I wrote about this once.
How one day, we'd scatter the map
living our own terribly separate lives
and how gently heartbreaking this would be,

that the progress to it crept so slow and silent
before we looked up and noticed the bulk of the years
wedged between.
I do hope you all know
how I could not have loved this place -

for Eleanor

how I could not have loved even myself -
my outstretched hands and their mercy cries -
without being loved by you.

Faded as the memories are,
decay creeps along the walls of so many buildings
here -
but never those where I knew you.

In the late nights and laughter.
In the spewing tears and early mornings,
where we loved so deeply and fully
for better and worse.

Where childhood ended like a thunderstorm
and you were the color in the sky.

for our tower and all that it birthed

for Eleanor

At the Newport

Injected into the crowd-
a room where I've been reborn
so many times.

Body hot with labor, I go
head first into the sticky abyss.

Lumbering, inexperienced into this void where I think
ought to be, and searching for the best place to land.

Every time, new skin under the lights.
Every time, new lights dancing across the belly of the
animal.

Always a fresh muse to carry me fearlessly into the
thick of it.

I am reincarnated once again.

for Eleanor

for Eleanor

On Spontaneity

Most of the time
I feel most intimate with strangers

going like air into some unsolved moment
and breathing into it answers of my own

that bend and shape
and reshape with the passing time.

Isn't everything most beautiful
when you first see it?

An innocent
unbitten by scorn.

Undulled by
that gray monotony

which rides in
covert

under the perfectly hemmed
cloak of consistency

draining the color
from the world.

I follow a butterfly through
the gate next door

boasting childlike wonder
in the name of Who Could've Been

for Eleanor

and in some chaotic anecdote
fed by impulse

a new life unfurls.
I swear

on all my breath
to make it a great one.

for Eleanor

The boy with a chest like a swallow finds it
and I stop writing alternate endings.
A scar across the face,
healed by some miracle.

Finally leaving home without the hat's brim low.
We have seen too much darkness
not to be in the bright now that we may.

Isn't it so beautiful, sometimes -
to close the book for good?

for Eleanor

for Eleanor

All Things Go

I told you once how this would happen.

When your father was still
strumming that acoustic
and my daughter danced
so intimately beneath my skin.

That day that I hoped the land line's crackle would
soothe in a time of grieving -
though not even death is as eerie quiet as
silence on the other end of an 'I love you.'

I told you, one day, when I was older, and I am,

I'd hold this town in my palm
the way you did - or the way I thought you did -
back before I had any smile lines and the top of your
hair thinned out so.

"This *will* disappear," I said.

"Your eyes to mine - all
you didn't know you needed -
I'll see windex on a glass door,
in some crowd, on some cool Ohio day."

And this afternoon
wasn't so chilly as expected,
but had a dove seen what i did
in looking at you, it may have been her last flight.

The breeze rustles the leaves.

for Eleanor

You read another poem.
And the one thing
this all reminds me of is

how sorrowfully you've always managed to smile.

for Eleanor

The Earth Cracks Open Again

Turns itself inside out -
becomes, as always, more enchanting-
more terrifying.

I stand, unafraid of the
knife - or the next battle.

Certain confidence - a calculated lack of faith in the
opponent.

Wouldn't you love to have me?
The woman who couldn't lose. The heavy hitter.

I could take whatever I want to
without remorse, I suppose.
Didn't I earn it after all these scars?

But I snap my fingers and the earth listens
My unbridled dreams
come quick and arrive panting

with eyes that apologize for taking so long.
How did I get here -
the bloody girl crying for a reason to stitch the wound?

for Eleanor

for Eleanor

Eleanor

Dear Eleanor,

I'll tell you a secret -
I haven't quite fixed myself
yet. Suspect it'll be a while
before I do.

Last week, I slept
through every morsel of
daylight - eyes bleary with saltwater
when they were open.

Hated myself for being so
broken while so fortunate.
Hated myself
but didn't mean it.
Hated myself-
until I remembered

You.
The spring that
burgeoned peace from careless soil.
The summer that
breathed color into paling skin.

The knowing that,
even before any of this,
autumn was always meant be
Ours.

You
and I

for Eleanor

and the long year's wavering tempo -

growing vibrant and strong
just in time to tumble back to earth,
becoming fuel for new
nourishment all over again.

Dear Eleanor,

Today, I wake
and leave the house-
a victory. To my surprise
the world is still
intact. Life

beyond the window -
laughter echoing through
quiet rooms.

Water, rushing down
rocks in races to the foothills,
and falling upon the flushed
cheeks of the heartbroken,

and sitting ever so still
in mossy quarries,
braced for impact
as young thrill seekers
leap from jagged cliffs above.

Lovers, losing each other.
Lovers finding each other again.
Passenger airplanes taking flight
while private jets touchdown.

for Eleanor

Children wailing in the grocery store
and adolescents skipping class to smoke weed
and grandparents, sat by landlines
on their birthdays in late afternoon -

and You -
with no chance
to see any of it.

I meant to compile scrolls
of lessons in these pages
for You, I swear. Wisdom
and certainty. Promises
and road maps -

all of which
evade my pen when
You are not here
to relay them to.

None of which
could bring your soft body
back into your mother's arms
with life enough
to learn them anyhow.

Dear Eleanor,

Leaves are crumbling
on the ground
again. Orange and red and
yellow under ever-earlier twilights.

for Eleanor

I resign
for the umpteenth time
to this reality -

that of us two,
the universe has not chosen me
to do the teaching.

Today I wake,
as yesterday - as the day before -
on behalf of Us both.

I still carve your name into
everything that is beautiful.

with all my love forever,
your mother.

for Eleanor

for Eleanor

for Eleanor

Thank you for reading!

For questions, commissions, more content, or to learn more about the poet, contact:

Laurendecamillo@gmail.com

@decam.writes on Instagram

for Eleanor